Delicious Slow Cooker

Recipes

Easy & Super Tasty Soups to Make

Unforgettable Lunch

Donna Conway

Table of Contents

Creamy Potato Soup

Preparation time: 15 minutes

Cooking time: 6 hours

Servings: 4 people

Ingredients:

- 6 slices of bacon, cut into 1/2-inch pieces

- 1 onion, finely chopped

- 2 (10.5 oz.) condensed chicken broth

- 2 cups of water

- 5 large potatoes, diced

- 1/2 teaspoon of salt

- 1/2 teaspoon dried dill weed

- 1/2 teaspoon ground white pepper

- 1/2 cup all-purpose flour

- 2 cups half and half cream

- 1 (12 fluid ounce) can evaporate milk

Directions:

1. Put bacon and onion in a large, deep frying pan. Bake over medium heat until the bacon is evenly browned and the onions are soft. Drain excess fat.

2. Transfer the bacon and onion to a slow cooker and stir in the chicken stock, water, potatoes, salt, dill-weed, and white pepper. Cover and cook on the layer for 6 to 7 hours, stirring occasionally.

3. In a small bowl, beat the flour and half and half. Stir the soup together with the evaporated milk. Cover and cook another 30 minutes before serving.

Nutrition: Calories: 553 Fat: 19.3g Carbs: 74.2g Protein: 22g

Split Pea Soup with Bacon & Hash Browns

Preparation time: 15 minutes

Cooking time: 8 hours

Servings: 4 people

Ingredients:

- 1/4-pound bacon, minced

- 1-pound split peas, rinsed

- 1/3 (20 oz.) package of frozen southern-style hash-brown potatoes

- 1 onion, minced

- 3 carrots, peeled and diced

- 3 ribs of celery, diced

- 2 cloves of garlic, finely chopped

- 1/8 teaspoon ground black pepper

- 1 pinch of red pepper flakes (optional)

- 8 cups chicken broth

Directions:

1. Put bacon in your large frying pan and cook over medium heat, occasionally turning, until light brown, about 5 minutes. Drain on kitchen paper.

2. Put bacon, split peas, baked potatoes, onion, carrots, celery, garlic, black pepper, red pepper flakes, and chicken broth in a slow cooker; stir to combine—Cook for 8 hours on low or high for 6 hours.

Nutrition: Calories: 258 Fat: 2.9g Carbs: 43g Protein: 16.7g

Southwest Black Bean Chicken Soup

Preparation time: 15 minutes

Cooking time: 8 hours

Servings: 4 people

Ingredients:

- 1 pound of cooked dark meat chicken

- 3 cans of black beans, rinsed

- 2 cans of chicken broth

- 2 cans tomatoes (diced) with green chili peppers

- 1 can of whole kernel corn

- ½ large onion, minced

- ½ cup chopped jalapeno peppers

- 2 cloves of garlic, minced

- 2 ½ teaspoons of chili powder

- 2 teaspoons of red pepper flakes

- 2 teaspoons of ground cumin

- 1 teaspoon ground coriander

- salt and ground black pepper to taste

- ½ cup sour cream, or to taste

Directions:

1. Put all fixing except for sour cream in a slow cooker; cook on low for 8 hours. Serve with about 1 tablespoon of sour cream on each serving.

Nutrition: Calories: 389 Fat: 13.1g Carbs: 43.7g Protein: 26.6g

Zucchini Soup

Preparation time: 15 minutes

Cooking time: 4 hours & 17 minutes

Servings: 4 people

Ingredients:

- 1 & 1/2 pounds sweet Italian sausage

- 1/2-inch pieces of celery

- 2-pound zucchini, cut into 1/2-inch slices

- 2 cans of tomatoes in cubes

- 2 green peppers, cut into 1/2-inch slices

- 1 cup chopped onion

- 2 teaspoons of salt

- 1 teaspoon of white sugar

- 1 teaspoon dried oregano

- 1 teaspoon of Italian herbs

- 1 teaspoon dried basil

- 1/4 teaspoon garlic powder

- 6 tablespoons grated Parmesan cheese, or to taste

Directions:

1. Heat-up a large frying pan over medium heat. Cook and stir sausage in the hot frying pan until brown and crumbly, 5 to 7 minutes; drain and throw away fat. Mix celery with cooked sausage; cook and stir until the celery is soft, about 10 minutes.

2. Combine sausage mix, zucchini, tomatoes, bell pepper, onion, salt, sugar, oregano, Italian herbs, basil, and garlic powder in a slow cooker. Cook on low within 4 to 6 hours. Garnish each portion with 1 tablespoon of parmesan cheese.

Nutrition: Calories: 389 Fat: 23.6g Carbs: 25.8 Protein: 21.8g

German Lentil Soup

Preparation time: 10 minutes

Cooking time: 8-10 hours

Servings: 4 people

Ingredients:

- 2 cups of dried brown lentils, rinsed and drained

- 3 cups of chicken broth

- 1 bay leaf

- 1 cup chopped carrots

- 1 cup chopped celery

- 1 cup chopped onion

- 1 cup of cooked, diced ham

- 1 teaspoon Worcestershire sauce

- 1/2 teaspoon of garlic powder

- 1/4 teaspoon freshly grated nutmeg

- 5 drops of hot pepper sauce

- 1/4 teaspoon caraway seeds

- 1/2 teaspoon celery salt

- 1 tablespoon chopped fresh parsley

- 1/2 teaspoon ground black pepper

Directions:

1. Place lentils in a slow cooker. Add chicken broth, bay leaves, carrots, celery, onion, and ham. Season with Worcestershire sauce, garlic powder, nutmeg, hot pepper sauce, caraway seeds, celery salt, parsley, and pepper. Cover and cook on low within 8 to 10 hours. Remove laurel before serving.

Nutrition: Calories: 221 Fat: 2.3 g Carbs: 34.2g

Protein: 16g

Chicken and Dumplings

Preparation time: 10 minutes

Cooking time: 6 hours

Servings: 4 people

Ingredients:

- 4 chicken fillets without skin, boneless

- 2 tablespoons butter

- 2 cans of condensed cream chicken soup

- 1 onion, finely chopped

- 2 packages of chilled biscuit dough, torn into pieces

Directions:

1. Place the chicken, butter, soup, and onion in a slow cooker and fill with enough water to cover.

2. Cover and cook on high within 5 to 6 hours. Place the cracked cookie dough in the slow cooker about 30 minutes before serving. Cook until the dough is no longer raw in the middle.

Nutrition:

Calories: 385

Fat: 18 g

Carbs: 37 g

Protein: 18.1 g

Chicken Taco Soup

Preparation time: 15 minutes

Cooking time: 7 hours

Servings: 4 people

Ingredients:

- 1 onion, minced

- 1 can of chili beans

- 1 can of black beans

- 1 can of whole kernel corn, drained

- 1 can of tomato sauce

- 1 can or bottle of beer

- 2 cans diced tomatoes with green peppers, undrained

- 1 taco herbs

- 3 whole chicken fillets without skin, without bones

- 8 oz grated cheddar cheese (optional)

- sour cream (optional)

- ground tortilla chips (optional)

Directions:

1. Put the onion, chili beans, black beans, corn, tomato sauce, beer, and diced tomatoes in a slow cooker. Add taco spices and stir to mix.

2. Place the chicken fillets on the mixture and press lightly until just covered with the other ingredients. Put the slow cooker on low heat, cover, and cook for 5 hours.

3. Remove the chicken fillets from the soup and let them cool for a long time to be handled. Stir the grated chicken back into the soup and continue to cook for 2 hours. Serve garnished with grated cheddar cheese, a dollop of sour cream, and possibly ground tortilla chips.

Nutrition:

Calories: 434

Fat: 17.7g

Carbs: 42.3g

Protein: 27.2g

Lentil and Ham Soup

Preparation time: 15 minutes

Cooking time: 11 hours

Servings: 4 people

Ingredients:

- 1 cup of dried lentils

- 1 cup chopped celery

- 1 cup chopped carrots

- 1 cup chopped onion

- 2 cloves of garlic, finely chopped

- 1 1/2 cups diced cooked ham

- 1/2 teaspoon dried basil

- 1/4 teaspoon dried thyme

- 1/2 teaspoon dried oregano

- 1 bay leaf

- 1/4 teaspoon of black pepper

- 32 grams of chicken broth

- 1 cup of water

- 8 teaspoons tomato sauce

Directions:

1. In a slow cooker, combine the lentils, celery, carrots, onion, garlic, and ham. Season with basil, thyme, oregano, bay leaf, and pepper.

2. Stir in the chicken stock, water, and tomato sauce—cover and cook on low for 11 hours. Discard the bay leaf before serving.

Nutrition: Calories: 222 Fat: 6.1g Carbs: 26.3g Protein: 15.1g

Cabbage Beef Soup

Preparation time: 15 minutes

Cooking time: 8 hours

Servings: 4 people

Ingredients:

- 2 tablespoons vegetable oil

- 1-pound ground beef

- 1/2 large onion, minced

- 5 cups chopped cabbage

- 2 (16 oz.) cans of red kidney beans, drained

- 2 cups of water

- 24 grams of tomato sauce

- 4 beef broth cubes

- 1 1/2 teaspoon ground cumin

- 1 teaspoon of salt

- 1 teaspoon pepper

Directions:

1. Heat oil in a large soup pot over medium heat. Add minced meat and onion and fry until the beef is well browned and crumbled.

2. Drain the fat and move the meat to a slow cooker. Add cabbage, kidney beans, water, tomato sauce, broth, cumin, salt, and pepper. Stir to dissolve broth and cover.

3. Cook for 4 hours on a high or low for 6 to 8 hours. Stir occasionally. To enjoy!

Nutrition: Calories: 211 Fat: 8.7g Carbs: 20.3g Protein: 14.1g

Split Pea Sausage Soup

Preparation time: 15 minutes

Cooking time: 5 hours

Servings: 4 people

Ingredients:

- 1 pound of dried split peas

- 10 cups of water

- 1 pound of smoked sausage of your choice, sliced

- 5 cubes of chicken broth

- 1 1/2 cups chopped carrot

- 1 cup chopped celery

- 2 potatoes, peeled and minced

- 1/2 teaspoon of garlic powder

- 1/2 teaspoon dried oregano

- 2 bay leaves

- 1 onion, minced

Directions:

1. In a slow cooker, combine the peas, water, sausage, broth, carrot, celery, potatoes, garlic powder, oregano, bay leaves, and onion. Cover and cook on high within 4 to 5 hours. Remove bay leaves before pouring them into bowls.

Nutrition:

Calories: 412

Fat: 13.1g

Carbs: 50.8g

Protein: 23.9g

Beef Vegetable Soup

Preparation time: 10 minutes

Cooking time: 6 hours

Servings: 4 people

Ingredients:

- 1-pound diced beef

- 1 can of whole kernel corn, undrained

- 1 can of green beans

- 1 can of carrots with juice

- 1 can of sliced potatoes with juice

- 1 can of crushed tomatoes

- 1 package of beef with onion soup mix

- salt and pepper to taste

Directions:

1. Put meat, corn, green beans, carrots, potatoes, tomatoes, soup mix, and salt and pepper to taste in the slow cooker; stir to combine. Cook on low for at least 6 hours. Add water if necessary.

Nutrition:

Calories: 364

Fat: 16.2g

Carbs: 38.8g

Protein: 20g

Spicy Black Bean Soup

Preparation time: 5 minutes

Cooking time: 5 hours

Servings: 4 people

Ingredients:

- 1 pound of dry black beans, soaked overnight, rinsed after

- 4 teaspoons diced jalapeno peppers

- 6 cups chicken broth

- 1/2 teaspoon of garlic powder

- 1 tbsp chili powder

- 1 tsp ground cumin

- 1 tsp cayenne pepper

- 3/4 tsp ground black pepper

- 1/2 tsp hot pepper sauce

Directions:

1. Mix beans, jalapenos, plus chicken broth in a slow cooker. Flavor it with garlic powder, chili powder, cumin, cayenne pepper, pepper, and hot pepper sauce.

2. Cook on high for 4 hours. Lower down the heat, then cook again within 2 hours or until you are ready to eat.

Nutrition:

Calories: 281

Fat: 2g

Carbs: 49.7g

Protein: 17.7g

Best Italian Sausage Soup

Preparation time: 15 minutes

Cooking time: 6 hours

Servings: 4 people

Ingredients:

- & 1/2-pounds Italian sausage, sweet

- 2 cloves of garlic, finely chopped

- 2 small onions, finely chopped

- 2 cans of whole peeled tomatoes

- 1 1/4 cups of red wine, dry

- 5 cups of beef broth

- 1/2 teaspoon dried basil

- 1/2 teaspoon dried oregano

- 2 courgettes, sliced

- 1 green pepper, minced

- 3 tablespoons chopped fresh parsley

- 1 package of spinach fettuccine pasta

- salt and pepper to taste

Directions:

1. Cook the sausage in your large saucepan on medium heat until brown. Remove with a spoon with a slot and drain on kitchen paper. Pour fat from the pan and save 3 tablespoons.

2. Cook garlic and onion in reserved fat for 2 to 3 minutes. Stir in tomatoes, wine, broth, basil, and oregano. Transfer to a slow cooker and stir in sausage, zucchini, pepper, and parsley. Cover and cook on low within 4 to 6 hours.

3. Bring a pot of lightly salted water to a boil. Cook the pasta in boiling water until al dente, about 7 minutes.

4. Drain water and add pasta to the slow cooker. Let simmer for a few minutes and season with salt and pepper before serving.

Nutrition:

Calories: 436

Fat: 17.8g

Carbs: 43.5g

Protein: 21g

Ham Bone Soup

Preparation time: 15 minutes

Cooking time: 6 hours

Servings: 4 people

Ingredients:

- 1 ham with some meat

- 1 onion, diced

- 1 can tomatoes with juice and diced

- 1 can of kidney beans

- 3 potatoes, diced

- 1 green pepper, without seeds and in cubes

- 4 cups of water

- 6 cubes of chicken broth

Directions:

1. Put the ham bone, onion, tomatoes, kidney beans, potatoes, plus green pepper in a slow cooker. Melt the bouillon cubes in water, then pour into the slow cooker. Cook on high until it is hot. Turn down the heat and cook for another 5 to 6 hours.

Nutrition:

Calories: 266

Fat: 1g

Carbs: 53.3g

Protein: 11.4g

Brussels Sprouts Soup

Preparation time: 5 minutes

Cooking time: 8 hours

Servings: 3 people

Ingredients:

- 1 lb. fresh brussels sprouts, halved

- 7 oz fresh baby spinach, torn

- 1 tsp of sea salt

- 1 cup of whole milk

- 3 tbsp of sour cream

- 1 tbsp of fresh celery, finely chopped

- 1 tsp of granulated sugar

- 2 cups of water

- 1 tbsp of butter

Directions:

1. Combine the ingredients in a slow cooker. Set the heat to low and cook for 8 hours. Open the cooker and transfer the soup to a food processor. Blend well to combine and serve.

Nutrition:

Calories: 194

Proteins 10g

Carbs: 21.7g

Fat: 9.8g

Classic Ragout Soup

Preparation time: 5 minutes

Cooking time: 8 hours

Servings: 4 people

Ingredients:

- 1 lb. lamb chops, 1 inch thick

- 1 cup of peas, rinsed

- 4 medium-sized carrots, peeled and finely chopped

- 3 small onions, peeled and finely chopped

- 1 large potato, peeled and finely chopped

- 1 large tomato, peeled and roughly chopped

- 3 tbsp of extra virgin olive oil

- 1 tbsp of cayenne pepper

- 1 tsp of salt

- ½ tsp of freshly ground black pepper

Directions:

1. Cut meat into bite-sized pieces. Make the first layer in your slow cooker. Now add peas, finely chopped carrots, onions, potatoes, and roughly chopped tomato.

2. Add about three tablespoons of olive oil, cayenne pepper, salt, and pepper. Give it a good stir and close the lid. Set for 8 hours on low.

Tip: If you have some spare time, try this simple trick to give your ragout an extra flavor. Heat-up 2-3 tablespoons of olive oil in a large skillet. Add meat chops and briefly brown on both sides. Transfer to a slow cooker and follow the recipe. Frying the meat just before cooking doesn't take more than five minutes and will give you an extra crispy flavor you simply can't get by just cooking.

Nutrition: Calories: 307 Proteins 24.9g Carbs: 23.3g Fat: 13g

Gorgonzola Broccoli Soup

Preparation time: 5 minutes

Cooking time: 2 hours

Servings: 4 people

Ingredients:

- 10 oz of Gorgonzola cheese, crumbled

- 1 cup of broccoli, finely chopped

- 1 tbsp of olive oil

- ½ cup of full-fat milk

- ½ cup of vegetable broth

- 1 tbsp of parsley, finely chopped

- ½ tsp of salt

- ¼ tsp of black pepper, ground

Directions:

1. Grease the bottom of a slow cooker with olive oil. Add all ingredients and three cups of water. Mix well with a kitchen whisker until thoroughly combined.

2. Cover with a lid and cook for 2 hours on low settings. Remove from the heat and sprinkle with some fresh parsley for extra taste.

Nutrition:

Calories: 208

Proteins 11.8g

Carbs: 7.6g

Fat: 15.8g

Moroccan Chickpea Soup

Preparation time: 15 minutes

Cooking time: 7 hours

Servings: 4 people

Ingredients:

- 14 oz chickpeas, soaked

- 2 large carrots, finely chopped

- 2 small onions, peeled and finely chopped

- 2 large tomatoes, peeled and finely chopped

- 3 tbsp of tomato paste

- A handful of fresh parsley, finely chopped

- 2 cups of vegetable broth

- 3 tbsp of extra virgin olive oil

- 1 tsp of salt

Directions:

1. Soak the chickpeas overnight. Rinse and drain. Set aside. Oiled bottom of your slow cooker with three tablespoons of olive oil. Place the rinsed chickpeas, chopped onions, carrots, and finely chopped tomatoes.

2. Pour the vegetable broth and season with salt. Stir in tomato paste and securely lock the lid. Set the heat to low and cook for 7 hours. Sprinkle with fresh parsley and serve.

Nutrition:

Calories: 420

Proteins 18.9g

Carbs: 58.6g

Fat: 14g

Pumpkin Soup

Preparation time: 5 minutes

Cooking time: 4 hours

Servings: 2 people

Ingredients:

- 2 lb. pumpkin, pureed

- 1 large onion, peeled and finely chopped

- 3 cups of vegetable broth

- 1 tbsp of ground turmeric

- ½ cup of double cream

- ½ tsp of salt

- A handful of fresh parsley

- 3 tbsp of extra virgin olive oil

Directions:

1. Place finely chopped onion, pureed pumpkin, turmeric, salt, and olive oil in your slow cooker. Add vegetable broth and stir well. Cover and set the heat to low. Cook for 4 hours.

2. Remove the lid, then stir in the double cream. Top with chopped parsley, then serve.

Nutrition:

Calories: 215

Proteins 5.6g

Carbs: 19.2g

Fat: 14.3g

Spring Spinach Soup

Preparation time: 15 minutes

Cooking time: 8 hours

Servings: 4 people

Ingredients:

- 1 lb. of lamb shoulder, cut into bite-sized pieces

- 12 oz fresh spinach leaves, torn

- 3 eggs, beaten

- 4 cups of vegetable broth

- 3 tbsp of extra virgin olive oil

- 1 tsp of salt

Directions:

1. Rinse and drain each spinach leaf. Cut into bite-sized pieces. Place in a slow cooker.

2. Sprinkle the meat generously with salt and transfer to a cooker, then put the other ingredients and whisk in three beaten eggs. Close the lid and cook for 8 hours on low.

Nutrition:

Calories: 325

Proteins 34.6g

Carbs: 3.4g

Fat: 19g

The Sultan's Soup

Preparation time: 10 minutes

Cooking time: 8 hours

Servings: 4 people

Ingredients:

- 3 1/2 oz of carrots, finely chopped

- 3 ½ oz of celery root, finely chopped

- A handful of green peas, soaked

- A handful of fresh okra

- 2 tbsp of butter

- 2 tbsp of fresh parsley, finely chopped

- 1 egg yolk

- 2 tbsp of cheese

- ¼ cup of freshly squeezed lemon juice

- 1 bay leaf

- 1 tsp of salt

- ½ tsp of pepper

- 4 cups of beef broth plus one cup of water

Directions:

1. Preparing this lovely soup in a slow cooker is very easy. Combine the ingredients in a slow cooker and close the lid. Set the heat to low and cook for 8 hours. Serve warm and enjoy!

Nutrition:

Calories: 161

Proteins 2.8g

Carbs: 9.1g

Fat: 13g

Bacon Chili

Preparation time: 15 minutes

Cooking time: 5 hours

Servings: 4 people

Ingredients:

- ½ tsp. pepper

- ¾ white onion

- 1 green bell pepper

- 1 Roma tomato

- 1 tbsp. chili powder

- 1 tsp. Worcestershire sauce

- 1 tsp. oregano

- 1 tsp. salt

- 2 cups chicken stock

- 2 jalapeno peppers

- 2 tsp. cumin

- 3 garlic cloves

- 30-oz. lean ground beef

- 5 slices of bacon

Directions:

1. Chop-up bacon, then adds to the pan. Cook until fat renders out, then the bacon is almost cooked. Then add beef to the pan, cooking till some color forms.

2. Chop up jalapeno peppers and garlic finely. Roughly chop up an onion, bell pepper, and tomato. Add 2 cups of stock to the slow cooker along with all other ingredients. Combine well.

3. Cook for 2 ½ hours on high or low for 5 hours. Serve.

Nutrition:

Calories: 527

Carbs: 7g

Fat: 37g

Protein: 51g

Steak Lover's Chili

Preparation time: 15 minutes

Cooking time: 6 hours

Servings: 4 people

Ingredients:

- ¼ tsp cayenne pepper

- ½ cup sliced leeks

- ½ tsp cumin

- ½ tsp salt

- 1 cup chicken stock

- 1 tbsp chili powder

- 1/8 tsp pepper

- 2 ½ pounds steak, sliced into 1-inch cubes

- 2 cups canned tomatoes

Optional Toppings:

- ¼ cup shredded cheddar cheese

- ½ sliced avocado

- 1 tsp. cilantro

- 2 tbsp. sour cream

Directions:

1. Pour all ingredients into your slow cooker, except topping components. Stir well to incorporate. Set to cook on high 6 hours. Shred cubes of steak and break up tomatoes. Serve topped with desired toppings.

Nutrition:

Calories: 198

Carbs: 6g

Fat: 19g

Protein: 11g

Buffalo Chicken Chili

Preparation time: 15 minutes

Cooking time: 8 hours

Servings: 4 people

Ingredients:

- ¼ - ½ cup buffalo wing sauce

- ¼ tsp. salt

- ½ tsp. celery salt

- ½ tsp. dried cilantro

- ½ tsp. garlic powder

- ½ tsp. onion powder

- 1 cup of frozen corn

- 1 package of ranch dressing mix

- 1-pound ground chicken

- 14 ½ ounce can fire-roasted tomatoes

- 15-ounce can white navy beans

- 2 cup chicken broth

- 8-oz. cream cheese

Directions:

1. Brown chicken in skillet till cooked. Place into the slow cooker. Mix in all remaining ingredients to chicken, mixing well to incorporate.

2. Cook within 4 hours on high or 8 hours on low. Stir well to incorporate cream cheese and wing sauce throughout the chili mixture.

Nutrition:

Calories: 277

Carbs: 11g

Fat: 14g

Protein: 17g

No Bean Chili

Preparation time: 15 minutes

Cooking time: 6-7 hours

Servings: 4 people

Ingredients:

- 1 cup of water
- 1 packet of chili seasoning
- 1 can dice tomatoes
- 1 can tomato sauce
- 2 pounds lean ground beef

Directions:

1. Cook ground beef and then add to slow cooker. Add the rest of your ingredients, stirring thoroughly to combine well.

2. Cook on low heat 6-7 hours. Serve topped with favorite toppings such as sour cream, cheese, diced onion, etc. Serve.

Nutrition:

Calories: 201

Carbs: 2g

Fat: 19g

Protein: 21g

Kickin' Chili

Preparation time: 15 minutes

Cooking time: 6-8 hours

Servings: 4 people

Ingredients:

- ¼ cup pickled jalapeno slices
- ½ tsp. cayenne pepper
- 1 bay leaf
- 1 chopped red onion
- 1 tsp. garlic powder
- 1 tsp. onion powder
- 1 tsp. oregano
- 1 tsp. pepper
- 14 ½ oz can stew tomatoes
- 14 ½ oz can tomato with green chilies
- 2 ½ pounds ground beef

- 2 tbsp. cumin

- 2 tbsp. Worcestershire sauce

- 2 tsp. salt

- 3 diced celery ribs

- 4 tbsp. chili powder

- 4 tbsp. minced garlic

- 6-ounce can tomato paste

Directions:

1. Turn the slow cooker to low. Brown beef in skillet along with pepper, salt, and 2 tablespoons of minced garlic. Drain excess grease.

2. Pour beef into the slow cooker. Add remaining recipe components and mix well. Cook 6-8 hours on low. Serve.

Nutrition: Calories: 137 Carbs: 5g Fat: 15g Protein: 16g

Creamy White Chicken Chili

Preparation time: 15 minutes

Cooking time: 7 hours

Servings: 4 people

Ingredients:

- ½ cup chicken stock
- ½ cup heavy cream
- ½ cup sour cream
- 1 tsp. cumin
- 1 tsp. garlic powder
- 2 pounds of chicken
- 2 tsp. chili powder
- 3 tbsp. butter
- 4-oz. cream cheese
- 9-oz. chopped green chilies

Toppings:

- 1 cup shredded pepper jack cheese

- 1/3 cup peeled and chopped red onion

- 1/3 cup chopped cilantro

Directions:

1. Place chicken in the slow cooker. Add green chilies, chicken stock, garlic powder, cumin, and chili powder to chicken.

2. Set to cook on low 7 hours. Before you plan to eat, heat sour cream, cream cheese, heavy cream, and butter together in a pan, stirring till smooth. Shred chicken.

3. Pour cream cheese mixture over chicken, combining well to incorporate. Sprinkle with pepper jack, red onion, and cilantro.

Nutrition: Calories: 486 Carbs: 6g Fat: 33g Protein: 39g

Old-Fashioned Low-Carb Chili

Preparation time: 15 minutes

Cooking time: 3 hours

Servings: 4 people

Ingredients:

- 1 ½ cup diced celery

- 1 cup beef broth

- 1 chopped yellow onion

- 1 tbsp. cumin

- 1 tsp. garlic powder

- 1 tsp. Italian seasoning

- 1 tsp. pepper

- 1 tsp. salt

- 14 ½ oz crush tomatoes

- 14 ½ oz dice tomatoes with green chilies

- 2-pounds lean ground beef

- 2 tbsp. crushed red pepper flakes

- 3 tbsp. chili powder

- 3 tbsp. minced garlic

- 6-oz. tomato paste

Directions:

1. Cook beef in a pan until browned and drain grease. Add garlic to the pan and sauté 60 seconds.

2. Place beef in the slow cooker. Add remaining ingredients to beef. Stir to combine well—Cook within 6 hours on low or 3 hours on high. Serve.

Nutrition:

Calories: 318

Carbs: 4g

Fat: 24g

Protein: 17g

Italian Veggie Dinner Casserole

Preparation time: 15 minutes

Cooking time: 8 hours & 20 minutes

Servings: 4 people

Ingredients:

- 1 can chickpeas, rinsed and drained

- 3 medium carrots, peeled and sliced

- 1 medium onion, chopped

- 1 can diced tomatoes with juice

- 2 garlic cloves, chopped finely

- 1 can Italian-style tomato paste

- 1 cup of water

- 2 tsp. sugar

- 1 tsp. Italian seasoning

- Salt

- ground black pepper, to taste

- 1½ cup frozen cut green beans, thawed

- 1 cup uncooked elbow macaroni
- ½ cup Parmesan cheese, shredded

Directions:

1. Put all the ingredients except for green beans, macaroni, and parmesan cheese and stir to combine in a slow cooker.

2. Set the slow cooker on low and cook, covered for about 6-8 hours. Uncover the slow cooker and stir in the green beans and macaroni.

3. Cook, covered for about 20 minutes on high. Top with cheese and serve hot.

Nutrition:

Calories: 506

Carbs: 87.1g

Protein: 25.7g

Fat: 8.4g

Familiar Mediterranean Dish

Preparation time: 15 minutes

Cooking time: 4 hours

Servings: 4 people

Ingredients:

- 2¼ cup unsalted vegetable broth

- 1½ cup uncooked quinoa, rinsed

- 1 (15½-oz.) can chickpeas, drained and rinsed

- 1 cup red onions, sliced

- 2 garlic cloves, minced

- 2½ tbsp. olive oil

- Salt, to taste

- 2 tsp. fresh lemon juice

- ½ cup roasted red bell peppers, drained and chopped

- 4 cup fresh baby arugula

- 12 kalamata olives, pitted and halved lengthwise

- 2 oz. feta cheese, crumbled

66

- 2 tbsp. fresh oregano, chopped

Directions:

1. In a slow cooker, place the broth, quinoa, chickpeas, onions, garlic, 1½ tsp. of the oil, and salt and stir to combine. Set the slow cooker on low and cook, covered for about 3-4 hours.

2. Meanwhile, in a bowl, add the lemon juice, remaining oil, and salt and mix well. Uncover the slow cooker and with a fork, fluff the quinoa mixture.

3. In the slow cooker, add the olive oil mixture, bell peppers, and arugula and gently combine. Over the pot for about 5 minutes before serving. Garnish with the olives, feta cheese, and oregano and serve.

Nutrition: Calories: 536 Carbs: 78.5g Protein: 23.2g Fat: 16.1g

Artichoke Pasta

Preparation time: 15 minutes

Cooking time: 8 hours

Servings: 4 people

Ingredients:

- 3 cans diced tomatoes with basil, oregano, and garlic

- 2 cans artichoke hearts, drained and quartered

- 6 garlic cloves, minced

- ½ cup whipping cream

- 12 oz. dried fettuccine pasta

- ¼ cup pimiento-stuffed green olives

- ¼ cup feta cheese, crumbled

Directions:

1. Drain the juices from two of the cans of diced

   tomatoes. In a greased slow cooker, place the drained

and undrained tomatoes alongside the artichoke hearts and garlic and mix well.

2. Set the slow cooker on low and cook, covered for about 6-8 hours. In a large pan of salted boiling water, cook the pasta for about 8-10 minutes or according to the package's directions.

3. Drain, then rinse under cold running water the pasta. Uncover the slow cooker and stir in the whipping cream.

4. Divide the pasta onto serving plates and top with artichoke sauce. Garnish with olives and cheese and serve.

Nutrition:

Calories: 479

Carbs: 82.2g

Protein: 20.8g

Fat: 10.4g

Veggie Lasagna

Preparation time: 15 minutes

Cooking time: 2 hours

Servings: 4 people

Ingredients:

- 1 package baby spinach, chopped roughly

- 3 large portobello mushroom caps, sliced thinly

- 1 small zucchini, sliced thinly

- 1 container part-skim ricotta cheese

- 1 large egg

- 1 can diced tomatoes

- 1 can of crushed tomatoes

- 3 garlic cloves, minced

- Pinch of red pepper flakes, crushed

- 15 uncooked whole-wheat lasagna noodles

- 3 cups part-skim mozzarella, shredded and divided

Directions:

1. Put the spinach, zucchini, ricotta cheese, and egg and mix well in a large bowl. In another bowl, add both cans of tomatoes with juice, garlic, and red pepper flakes and mix well.

2. In the bottom of a generously greased slow cooker, place about 1½ cup of the tomato mixture evenly. Place 5 lasagna noodles over the tomato mixture, overlapping them slightly and breaking them to fit in the pot.

3. Put half of the ricotta batter over the noodles. Now, place about 1½ cup of the tomato mixture and sprinkle with 1 cup of the mozzarella. Repeat the layers twice.

4. Cook, covered for about 2 hours on high. Uncover the slow cooker and sprinkle with the remaining mozzarella cheese. Immediately cover the cooker for about 10 minutes before serving.

Nutrition: Calories: 289 Carbs: 37.1g Protein: 18.8g Fat: 8.2g

Homemade Hummus

Preparation time: 15 minutes

Cooking time: 4 hours

Servings: 4 people

Ingredients:

- 1½ cup dried chickpeas, rinsed

- 2-3 cups of water

- 2 garlic cloves, peeled

- ¼ cup olive oil

- 2 tbsp. fresh lemon juice

- ¼ cup tahini

Directions:

1. In a slow cooker, place the chickpeas and water. Set the slow cooker on high and cook, covered for about 4 hours.

2. Uncover the slow cooker, drain the chickpeas, reserve about 1/3 cup of the cooking liquid cooking and remaining ingredients, and pulse until smooth. Transfer the hummus into a bowl and refrigerator before serving.

Nutrition:

Calories: 190

Carbs: 19.7g

Protein: 6.9g

Fat: 10.1g

Barbecue Kabocha Squash

Preparation time: 15 minutes

Cooking time: 6-8 hours

Servings: 2 people

Ingredients:

- 1 teaspoon extra-virgin olive oil
- ½ kabocha squash, seeded, peeled, and cut into 2-by-1-inch pieces
- 1 red onion, halved and sliced thin
- 1 small sweet potato, cut into 1-inch pieces
- 1 cup tomato sauce
- ½ cup low-sodium vegetable broth
- 1 teaspoon Dijon mustard
- 1 teaspoon smoked paprika
- 1 teaspoon garlic powder
- 1 teaspoon onion powder
- 1 teaspoon maple syrup or honey

- 1/8 teaspoon sea salt

Directions:

1. Oiled inside of the slow cooker with olive oil. Put the squash, red onion, and sweet potato into the slow cooker.

2. In a small bowl, whisk together the tomato sauce, vegetable broth, mustard, paprika, garlic powder, onion powder, maple syrup, and salt. Pour this mixture over the vegetables.

3. Cover and cook on low within 6 to 8 hours, or until the squash is very tender.

Nutrition:

Calories: 236

Fat: 0g

Carbs: 48g

Protein: 7g

Braised Quinoa, Kale & Summer Squash

Preparation time: 10 minutes

Cooking time: 4 hours

Servings: 2 people

Ingredients:

- ½ cup quinoa

- ½ cup canned chickpeas drained and rinsed

- 1 cup diced summer squash

- 4 cups fresh kale

- 1 cup canned plum tomatoes, roughly chopped

- 2 cups low-sodium vegetable broth

- 1 tablespoon Italian herb blend

- 1/8 teaspoon sea salt

Directions:

1. Put all the fixings into the slow cooker, stirring to mix them thoroughly. Cover and cook on low within 4 hours.

Nutrition:

Calories: 342

Fat: 1g

Carbs: 56g

Protein: 19g

Rosemary Cauliflower & Lentils

Preparation time: 10 minutes

Cooking time: 8 hours

Servings: 2 people

Ingredients:

- 1 cup cauliflower florets

- 1 cup lentils

- 1 tablespoon fresh rosemary

- 1 tablespoon roasted garlic

- Zest of 1 lemon

- 1 tablespoon extra-virgin olive oil

- 1/8 teaspoon sea salt

- Freshly ground black pepper

- 3 cups low-sodium vegetable broth

- Juice of 1 lemon

- ¼ cup roughly chopped fresh parsley

Directions:

1. Put the cauliflower, lentils, rosemary, garlic, lemon zest, and olive oil in the slow cooker. Season with salt and black pepper.

2. Pour the vegetable broth over the cauliflower and lentils. Cover and cook on low within 8 hours. Before serving, drizzle the cauliflower and lentils with lemon juice and sprinkle the parsley over the top.

Nutrition:

Calories: 484

Fat: 2g

Carbs: 65g

Protein: 34g

Mixed Bean Chili

Preparation time: 10 minutes

Cooking time: 6-8 hours

Servings: 2 people

Ingredients:

- 1 (16-ounce) can mixed beans, drained and rinsed
- 1 cup frozen roasted corn kernels, thawed
- 1 cup canned fire-roasted diced tomatoes, undrained
- ½ cup diced onion
- 2 garlic cloves, minced
- 1 teaspoon ground cumin
- 1 teaspoon smoked paprika
- 1 teaspoon dried oregano
- 1/8 teaspoon sea salt

Directions:

1. Put all the ingredients in the slow cooker. Give them a quick stir to combine. Cover and cook on low within 6 to 8 hours. Serve.

Nutrition:

Calories: 257

Fat: 0g

Carbs: 58g

Protein: 13g

Curried Sweet Potatoes with Broccoli & Cashews

Preparation time: 15 minutes

Cooking time: 6-8 hours

Servings: 2 people

Ingredients:

- 2 medium sweet potatoes, cut into 1-inch pieces
- 1 cup broccoli florets
- ½ cup diced onions
- 1 cup light coconut milk
- 1 teaspoon minced fresh ginger
- 1 teaspoon minced garlic
- Pinch red pepper flakes
- 1 tablespoon curry powder
- 1 teaspoon garam masala
- ¼ cup toasted cashews

Directions:

1. Put the sweet potatoes, broccoli, and onions into the slow cooker. Mix the coconut milk, ginger, garlic, red pepper flakes, curry powder, and garam masala in a small bowl. Pour this mixture over the vegetables.

2. Cover and cook on low within 6 to 8 hours until the vegetables are very tender but not falling apart. Just before serving, add the cashews and stir thoroughly.

Nutrition:

Calories: 582

Fat: 27g

Carbs: 60g

Protein: 10g

Moroccan-Style Chickpeas with Chard

Preparation time: 15 minutes

Cooking time: 8 hours

Servings: 2 people

Ingredients:

- ½ bunch Swiss chard stems diced and leaves roughly chopped

- 1 (16-ounce) can chickpeas, drained and rinsed

- ½ cup diced onion

- ½ cup diced carrots

- ¼ cup diced dried apricots

- 2 tablespoons roughly chopped preserved lemons (optional)

- 1 tablespoon tomato paste

- 1 teaspoon minced fresh ginger

- ¼ teaspoon red pepper flakes

- ½ teaspoon smoked paprika

- ½ teaspoon ground cinnamon

- ¼ teaspoon ground cumin

- 1/8 teaspoon sea salt

Directions:

1. Put all the fixings into the slow cooker. Stir everything together thoroughly. Cover and cook on low within 8 hours. Serve.

Nutrition:

Calories: 84

Fat: 0g

Carbs: 17g

Protein: 4g

4 Spinach & Black Bean Enchilada Pie

Preparation time: 15 minutes

Cooking time: 6-8 hours

Servings: 2 people

Ingredients:

- 1 (15-ounce) can black beans, drained and rinsed
- ¼ cup low-fat cream cheese
- ¼ cup low-fat Cheddar cheese
- ½ cup minced onion
- 1 teaspoon minced garlic
- 1 teaspoon ground cumin
- 1 teaspoon smoked paprika
- 2 cups shredded fresh spinach
- 1 teaspoon extra-virgin olive oil
- 1 cup enchilada sauce, divided
- 4 corn tortillas

- ¼ cup fresh cilantro, for garnish

Directions:

1. Mix the beans, cream cheese, Cheddar cheese, onion, garlic, cumin, paprika, and spinach in a large bowl. Oiled inside of the slow cooker with olive oil.

2. Pour ¼ cup of enchilada sauce into the slow, spreading it across the bottom. Place one corn tortilla on top of the sauce, then top the tortilla with one-third of the black bean and spinach mixture.

3. Top this with a second corn tortilla, and then slather it with ¼ cup of enchilada sauce. Repeat this layering, finishing with a corn tortilla and the last ¼ cup of enchilada sauce.

4. Cover and cook on low within 6 to 8 hours. Garnish with the cilantro just before serving.

Nutrition: Calories: 373 Fat: 10g Carbs: 42g Protein: 13g

Spinach, Mushroom & Swiss Cheese Crustless Quiche

Preparation time: 10 minutes

Cooking time: 8 hours

Servings: 2 people

Ingredients:

- 1 teaspoon butter, at room temperature, or extra-virgin olive oil

- 4 eggs

- 1 teaspoon fresh thyme

- 1/8 teaspoon sea salt

- Freshly ground black pepper

- 2 slices whole-grain bread, crusts removed, cut into 1-inch cubes

- ½ cup diced button mushrooms

- 2 tablespoons minced onion

- 1 cup shredded spinach

- ½ cup shredded Swiss cheese

Directions:

1. Oiled inside of the slow cooker with the butter. In a small bowl, whisk together the eggs, thyme, salt, and a few black pepper grinds.

2. Put the bread, mushrooms, onions, spinach, and cheese in the slow cooker. Pour the egg mixture over the top and stir gently to combine. Cover and cook on low within 8 hours or overnight.

Nutrition:

Calories: 348

Saturated Fat: 9g

Carbs: 21g

Protein: 24g

Seitan Tikka Masala

Preparation time: 10 minutes

Cooking time: 6 hours

Servings: 2 people

Ingredients:

- 8 oz. seitan, cut into bite-size pieces

- 1 cup chopped green beans

- 1 cup diced onion

- 1 cup fire-roasted tomatoes, drained

- 1 teaspoon ground coriander

- 1 teaspoon ground cumin

- 1 teaspoon smoked paprika

- 1/8 teaspoon red pepper flakes

- 1 teaspoon minced fresh ginger

- 1 cup low-sodium vegetable broth

- 2 tablespoons coconut cream

- ¼ cup minced fresh cilantro, for garnish

Directions:

1. Put the seitan, green beans, onion, tomatoes, coriander, cumin, paprika, red pepper flakes, ginger, and vegetable broth in the slow cooker. Gently stir the ingredients together to combine.

2. Cover and cook on low within 6 hours. Allow the dish to rest, uncovered, for 10 minutes, then stir in the coconut cream and garnish the dish with the cilantro.

Nutrition:

Calories: 245

Fat: 3g

Carbs: 24g

Protein: 4g

Butter Seitan & Chickpeas

Preparation time: 15 minutes

Cooking time: 6-8 hours

Servings: 2 people

Ingredients:

- 1 teaspoon extra-virgin olive oil

- 8 oz. seitan, cut into bite-size pieces

- 1 (15-ounce) can chickpeas, drained and rinsed

- ½ cup minced onion

- 1 teaspoon minced garlic

- 2 tablespoons tomato paste

- 1 teaspoon minced fresh ginger

- ½ teaspoon garam masala

- 1 teaspoon curry powder

- Pinch red pepper flakes

- ½ teaspoon of sea salt

- 1 cup light coconut milk

Directions:

1. Oiled inside of the slow cooker with olive oil. Put all the fixings into the slow cooker and stir to mix thoroughly. Cover and cook on low within 6 to 8 hours.

Nutrition:

Calories: 302

Fat: 12g

Carbs: 17g

Protein: 4g

Tempeh Shepherd's Pie

Preparation time: 10 minutes

Cooking time: 8 hours

Servings: 2 people

Ingredients:

- 1 cup frozen peas, thawed

- 1 cup diced carrots

- ½ cup minced onions

- 8 oz. tempeh

- 1/8 teaspoon sea salt

- Freshly ground black pepper

- 1½ cups prepared mashed potatoes

- 2 tablespoons shredded sharp Cheddar cheese

Directions:

1. Put the peas, carrots, onions, and tempeh in the slow cooker and gently stir to combine. Season the batter with the salt plus black pepper.

2. Spread the prepared mashed potatoes over the tempeh and vegetable mixture. Cover and cook on low within 8 hours. Sprinkle with the cheese just before serving.

Nutrition:

Calories: 476

Fat: 6g

Carbs: 53g

Protein: 32g

Tempeh-Stuffed Bell Peppers

Preparation time: 10 minutes

Cooking time: 6-8 hours

Servings: 2 people

Ingredients:

- 1 teaspoon extra-virgin olive oil
- 8 oz. tempeh, crumbled
- 1 cup frozen corn kernels, thawed
- ¼ cup minced onions
- 1 teaspoon minced garlic
- 1 teaspoon ground cumin
- 1 teaspoon smoked paprika
- 2 tablespoons pepper Jack cheese
- 1/8 teaspoon sea salt
- 4 narrow red bell peppers

Directions:

1. Oiled inside of the slow cooker with olive oil. In a medium bowl, combine the tempeh, corn, onions, garlic, cumin, paprika, cheese, and salt.

2. Cut the tops off each of the peppers and set the tops aside. Scoop out and discard the seeds and membranes from inside each pepper. Divide the tempeh filling among the peppers. Return the tops to each of the peppers.

3. Nestle the peppers into the slow cooker. Cover and cook on low within 6 to 8 hours, until the peppers are very tender.

Nutrition:

Calories: 422

Fat: 5g

Carbs: 44g

Protein: 28g

Tofu Red Curry with Green Beans

Preparation time: 10 minutes

Cooking time: 6 hours

Servings: 2 people

Ingredients:

- 1 teaspoon extra-virgin olive oil

- 16 oz firm tofu, cut into 1-inch pieces

- 2 cups chopped green beans

- ½ red onion halved and sliced thin

- 1 plum tomato, diced

- 1 teaspoon minced fresh ginger

- 1 teaspoon minced garlic

- 2 teaspoons Thai red curry paste

- 1 cup of coconut milk

- 1 cup low-sodium vegetable broth

Directions:

1. Oiled inside of the slow cooker with olive oil. Put all the ingredients into the slow cooker, and stir gently. Cover and cook on low within 6 hours.

Nutrition:

Calories: 538

Fat: 28g

Carbs: 25g

Protein: 25g

Tofu Stir-Fry

Preparation time: 10 minutes

Cooking time: 4-6 hours

Servings: 2 people

Ingredients:

- 1 teaspoon extra-virgin olive oil

- ½ cup of brown rice

- 1 cup of water

- Pinch sea salt

- 1 (16-ounce) block tofu, drained and cut into 1-inch pieces

- 1 green bell pepper, cored and cut into long strips

- ½ onion halved and thinly sliced

- 1 cup chopped green beans, cut into 1-inch pieces

- 2 carrots, cut into ½-inch dice

- 2 tablespoons low-sodium soy sauce

- 1 tablespoon hoisin sauce

- 1 tablespoon freshly squeezed lime juice

- 1 teaspoon minced garlic

- Pinch red pepper flakes

Directions:

1. Oiled inside of the slow cooker with olive oil. Put the brown rice, water, and salt in the slow cooker and gently stir, so all the rice grains are submerged. Put the tofu, bell pepper, onion, green beans, and carrots over the rice.

2. In a measuring cup or glass jar, whisk together the soy sauce, hoisin sauce, lime juice, garlic, and red pepper flakes. Pour this batter over the tofu and vegetables.

3. Cover and cook on low for 4 to 6 hours, until the rice, has soaked up all the liquid and the vegetables are tender.

Nutrition: Calories: 456 Fat: 3g Carbs: 63g Protein: 26g

Spicy Peanut Rice Bake

Preparation time: 10 minutes

Cooking time: 6-8 hours

Servings: 2 people

Ingredients:

- 1 teaspoon extra-virgin olive oil

- ½ cup of brown rice

- 3 cups low-sodium vegetable broth, divided

- 4 collard leaves, ribs removed, chopped into thin ribbons

- ½ cup minced red onion

- 1 tablespoon minced ginger

- 2 tablespoons tomato paste

- ¼ cup unsalted creamy peanut butter

- 1 teaspoon Sriracha

- 1/8 teaspoon sea salt

- ¼ cup roughly chopped cilantro, for garnish

- Lime wedges, for garnish

- 2 tablespoons roasted peanuts, roughly chopped, for garnish

Directions:

1. Oiled inside of the slow cooker with olive oil. Put the rice, 2 cups of broth, collard greens, and onion in the slow cooker.

2. In a medium bowl, whisk together the remaining 1 cup of broth, ginger, tomato paste, peanut butter, Sriracha, and salt. Stir this mixture into the slow cooker.

3. Cover and cook on low within 6 to 8 hours. Garnish each serving with fresh cilantro, a lime wedge, and the peanuts. Serve.

Nutrition: Calories: 554 Fat: 13g Carbs: 59g Protein: 24g

Squash and Zucchini Casserole

Preparation time: 10 minutes

Cooking time: 6 hours

Servings: 4 people

Ingredients:

- 2 cups yellow squash, quartered and sliced

- 2 cups zucchini, quartered and sliced

- 1/4 cup Parmesan cheese, grated

- 1/4 cup butter, cut into pieces

- 1 tsp garlic powder

- 1 tsp Italian seasoning

- 1/4 tsp pepper

- 1/2 tsp sea salt

Directions:

1. Add sliced yellow squash and zucchini to a slow cooker. Sprinkle with garlic powder, Italian seasoning, pepper, and salt.

2. Top with grated cheese and butter. Cover with the lid and cook on low for 6 hours. Serve and enjoy.

Nutrition:

Calories: 107

Fat: 9.5g

Carbs: 2.5g

Protein: 2.6g

Almond Green Beans

Preparation time: 10 minutes

Cooking time: 3 hours

Servings: 4 people

Ingredients:

- 1 lb. green beans, rinsed and trimmed

- 1/2 cup almonds, sliced and toasted

- 1 cup vegetable stock

- 1/4 cup butter, melted

- 6 oz onion, sliced

- 1 tbsp olive oil

- 1/4 tsp pepper

- 1/2 tsp salt

Directions:

1. Heat-up olive oil in a pan over medium heat. Add onion to the pan and sauté until softened. Transfer sautéed onion to a slow cooker.

2. Add remaining ingredients except for almonds to the slow cooker and stir well. Cover and cook on low within 3 hours. Top with toasted almonds and serve.

Nutrition:

Calories: 253

Fat: 21.6g

Carbs: 14.5g

Protein: 5.1g

Ranch Mushrooms

Preparation time: 10 minutes

Cooking time: 3 Hours

Servings: 4 people

Ingredients:

- 2 lb. mushrooms, rinsed, pat dry

- 2 packets ranch dressing mix

- 3/4 cup butter, melted

- 1/4 cup fresh parsley, chopped

Directions:

1. Add all ingredients except parsley to a slow cooker and stir well. Cover and cook on low within 3 hours. Garnish with parsley and serve.

Nutrition: Calories: 237 Fat: 23.5g Carbs: 5.2g Protein: 5.1g

www.ingramcontent.com/pod-product-compliance
Lightning Source LLC
Chambersburg PA
CBHW071109030426
42336CB00013BA/2019